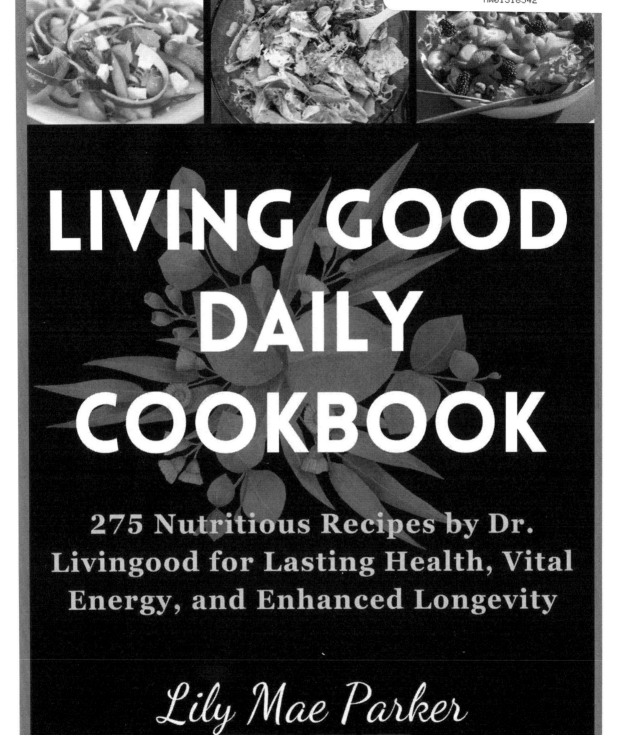

# LIVING GOOD DAILY COOKBOOK

### 275 Nutritious Recipes by Dr. Livingood for Lasting Health, Vital Energy, and Enhanced Longevity

*Lily Mae Parker*

Copyright © 2024 by Lily Mae Parker

**All rights reserved.**

No part of this book may be reproduced, distributed, or transmitted in any form or by any means, including photocopying, recording, or other electronic or mechanical methods, without the prior written permission of the publisher, except in the case of brief quotations embodied in critical reviews and certain other noncommercial uses permitted by copyright law.

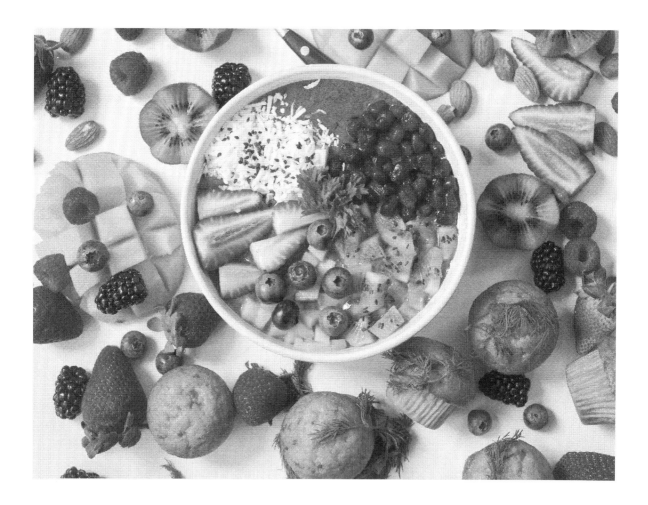

# Table of Contents

**Introduction: Redefining Health and Wellness**..........................7
  The Sick Care System vs. True Health Care...................9
  Why Food is Our Best Medicine...................10
  Building Health from the Inside Out...................11

**Chapter 1: Essentials for Living Good Daily**..........................14
  Foundational Principles of Real Health...................14
  Nutritional Basics for Disease Prevention...................17
  The Benefits of Whole Foods and Natural Ingredients...............19

**Chapter 2: Meal Planning for Lasting Health**..........................22
  Building a Balanced Meal Plan...................22
  Tips for Preparing Real Foods with Ease...................24
  Creating Weekly Meal Planning Templates and Shopping Lists. 26

**Chapter 3: Health-Building Breakfasts**..........................29
  Blueberry Chia Seed Pudding...................29
  Greek Yoghourt Parfait with Mixed Berries and Nuts...................30
  Avocado Toast with Egg...................31
  Overnight Oats with Banana and Almond Butter...................32
  Veggie-Packed Breakfast Burrito...................33
  Banana Spinach Smoothie...................34
  Quinoa Breakfast Bowl...................35
  Sweet Potato Hash with Eggs...................36
  Cottage Cheese with Pineapple and Flaxseed...................37
  Oatmeal with Almonds and Apples...................38
  Buckwheat Pancakes with Berries...................39
  Savory Oatmeal with Spinach and Feta...................40

Protein-Packed Smoothie Bowl..............................................................41

Apple Cinnamon Quinoa Bowl...............................................................42

Peanut Butter Banana Overnight Oats...................................................43

**Chapter 4: Nourishing Lunches for Sustained Energy............... 44**

Quinoa Salad with Chickpeas and Spinach........................................... 44

Turkey and Avocado Wrap..................................................................... 45

Mediterranean Grain Bowl..................................................................... 46

Sweet Potato and Black Bean Tacos.....................................................47

Lentil Soup with Carrots and Celery..................................................... 48

Chickpea and Avocado Salad................................................................ 49

Brown Rice Stir-Fry with Tofu............................................................... 50

Egg Salad Sandwich................................................................................51

Zucchini Noodles with Pesto and Cherry Tomatoes.......................... 52

Shrimp and Avocado Salad....................................................................53

Roasted Vegetable and Hummus Wrap...............................................54

Tuna Salad with Beans and Corn.......................................................... 55

Mushroom and Spinach Quinoa Bowl................................................. 56

Baked Falafel with Tahini Sauce...........................................................57

Cottage Cheese Bowl with Fruits and Nuts........................................ 58

**Chapter 5: Dinners that Heal and Restore....................................59**

Lemon Herb Grilled Chicken with Quinoa Salad.........................59

Baked Salmon with Sweet Potato and Asparagus..................... 60

Vegetable Stir-Fry with Brown Rice..................................................... 61

Quinoa-Stuffed Bell Peppers................................................................ 62

Lentil and Spinach Soup........................................................................ 63

Zucchini Noodles with Tomato Basil Sauce........................................64

Chickpea Curry with Brown Rice.......................................................... 65

Stuffed Acorn Squash.............................................................................66

Baked Eggplant Parmesan.................................................................... 67

Turkey and Vegetable Skillet.................................................................68

Mushroom and Spinach Risotto..................................................69
Honey-Garlic Shrimp with Broccoli..........................................70
Pasta Primavera.......................................................................71
Cauliflower Fried Rice.............................................................72
Balsamic Glazed Brussels Sprouts and Carrots.......................73

**Chapter 6: Desserts and Snacks for Real Health....................74**
Chia Seed Pudding...................................................................74
Avocado Chocolate Mousse....................................................75
Oatmeal Energy Bites..............................................................76
Banana Ice Cream....................................................................77
Almond Flour Chocolate Chip Cookies..................................78
Greek Yoghourt Parfait...........................................................79
Coconut Macaroons................................................................80
Sweet Potato Brownies...........................................................81
Berry Coconut Popsicles........................................................82
Dark Chocolate Dipped Fruit.................................................83
Pumpkin Spice Energy Bites..................................................84
Lemon Almond Energy Balls.................................................85
Apple Nachos..........................................................................86
Nut Butter Banana Bites........................................................87
Homemade Granola Bars......................................................88

**Chapter 7: Supercharged Smoothies and Juices..................89**
Green Power Smoothie..........................................................89
Berry Blast Smoothie.............................................................90
Tropical Mango Smoothie.....................................................91
Chocolate Peanut Butter Smoothie......................................92
Avocado Spinach Smoothie...................................................93
Cucumber Mint Juice.............................................................94
Beetroot Berry Smoothie......................................................95
Pineapple Green Juice...........................................................96

Coconut Banana Smoothie................................................................97

Carrot Ginger Juice........................................................................ 98

Orange Turmeric Smoothie..........................................................99

Apple Cinnamon Smoothie..........................................................100

Spinach Avocado Smoothie.......................................................... 101

Strawberry Basil Juice.................................................................. 102

Peach Green Smoothie................................................................. 103

## Chapter 8: 30-Day Meal Plan (Bonus 1)................................... 104

Day 1 to 7........................................................................................ 104

Day 8 to 14......................................................................................106

Day 15 to 21.................................................................................... 108

Day 22 to 30....................................................................................110

## Conclusion: Living Good Daily Beyond the Kitchen..................112

Healthy Habits for a Lifetime....................................................... 112

The Mind-Body Connection in Health........................................114

Encouragement for the Health-Building Journey....................115

## 4 BOOKS BONUS GIFTS.................................................................116

# Introduction: Redefining Health and Wellness

Imagine this: you're sitting in a doctor's office, feeling run-down, fatigued, or maybe struggling with chronic pain. You think back to the days when you felt vibrant, energetic, and fully alive. Somewhere along the way, that vitality faded. Your doctor looks at a chart, glances up, and tells you that medication might be necessary—perhaps for the rest of your life. A prescription is handed over, and in that moment, you realize that "health" as you once knew it has been redefined. You're no longer healthy; you're managing symptoms. Sound familiar?

This is the daily reality for millions of people. In the United States alone, we consume 75% of the world's medications. Seven out of ten people will die from chronic, preventable diseases, all while the very system meant to heal us—our healthcare system—is now the third leading cause of death itself. We are taught to assume that we're healthy until disease or chronic conditions suddenly make us feel otherwise. But what if we've been looking at health all wrong? What if the true solution lies not in managing sickness, but in actively building health?

This is what the LIVING GOOD DAILY COOKBOOK is all about. Unlike the countless diets, medications, and treatments that react to illness, this book gives you the tools to proactively create health from within, one meal at a time. Here, we break away from the band-aid solutions that treat symptoms and focus instead on sustainable, delicious, and simple recipes that transform your kitchen into a foundation of real, lasting health.

In these pages, you'll discover breakfasts that invigorate, lunches that keep you sharp and energised, dinners that restore, and snacks and drinks that are as nourishing as they are enjoyable.

Every recipe is crafted to help you make food your most powerful medicine, bringing vitality, energy, and resilience back into your life without complicated steps or hard-to-find ingredients. Whether you want to reduce inflammation, balance blood sugar, boost immunity, or simply feel alive again, the solutions are here, and they're simpler than you might think.

So, let's turn the page and take a stand for real health together. This book isn't just a collection of recipes—it's a blueprint for building a life of vitality, longevity, and joy, one meal at a time. Welcome to the journey of living good daily.

# The Sick Care System vs. True Health Care

In the world today, our healthcare system is heavily geared towards managing sickness rather than cultivating health. It's an approach often described as a "sick care system," where the primary focus is on identifying and treating symptoms of illness, often through medications or surgeries. This system has made impressive advances in treating acute diseases and life-threatening emergencies, but when it comes to chronic illnesses—such as heart disease, diabetes, and obesity—the approach falls short. Instead of addressing the root causes of these conditions, the sick care system often provides temporary fixes that mask symptoms rather than creating lasting health.

This reliance on a sick care system has made it one of the leading causes of death in the United States. Treatments often include medications with side effects, surgeries that require significant recovery, and lifestyle changes that many patients struggle to maintain. In this system, health is rarely defined as the presence of vitality and resilience; it's simply the absence of diagnosed disease. People often wait until something goes wrong before they make adjustments, and by then, years of poor lifestyle choices may have already taken their toll.

True health care, in contrast, is a proactive and preventative approach that nurtures and protects the body's natural resilience. It's built on the foundation that wellness is not merely about avoiding illness but actively creating conditions where disease has no place to grow. True health care takes into account lifestyle choices, diet, mental wellness, and overall well-being as the pillars of a healthy life. This approach looks at the whole person, focusing on the root causes of disease, such as inflammation, hormonal imbalances, and nutrient deficiencies, and uses them as starting points for building a better, healthier life.

# Why Food is Our Best Medicine

One of the most powerful tools for building true health is something we encounter every day: food. Since ancient times, various cultures have regarded food as medicine, and modern science supports this wisdom. The food we eat provides essential nutrients, fuels our cells, and interacts with our genes in complex ways that shape our overall health. Eating whole, natural foods can help reduce inflammation, boost immune function, stabilise blood sugar levels, and improve digestion—all vital elements for preventing and managing chronic disease.

The concept of food as medicine means understanding that what we eat can either contribute to health or undermine it. Processed foods loaded with sugars, unhealthy fats, and preservatives may offer convenience and flavor, but they deprive our bodies of the nutrients we need to thrive. These foods are often empty calories that fuel cravings, weaken immunity, and contribute to long-term health issues like obesity, heart disease, and even some forms of cancer.

In contrast, whole foods such as fresh vegetables, fruits, whole grains, and lean proteins are packed with the vitamins, minerals, fiber, and antioxidants that keep us vibrant. Cruciferous vegetables like broccoli and kale, for example, contain compounds that help detoxify the body, while berries provide antioxidants that combat oxidative stress. Lean proteins, such as those found in fish, eggs, and legumes, support muscle repair and metabolic health. Healthy fats, such as those in avocados, nuts, and olive oil, nourish the brain, help regulate hormones, and reduce inflammation.

By adopting a food-as-medicine mindset, we start to view each meal as an opportunity to invest in our health. We move away from calorie-counting or restrictive diets and instead focus on the quality of what we eat. With food as medicine, the emphasis shifts from deprivation to nourishment, from managing symptoms to creating balance.

This approach not only helps us address existing health concerns but also enables us to feel energetic, focused, and resilient—qualities that build a solid foundation for long-term health.

## Building Health from the Inside Out

Building health from the inside out requires adopting a mindset that focuses on prevention, nourishment, and sustainable habits. This approach goes beyond simply eliminating unhealthy foods; it's about nourishing the body, mind, and spirit to create a well-rounded state of wellness that can weather life's challenges.

**Focusing on Gut Health**

Gut health is foundational to overall wellness. The digestive system is responsible for breaking down food, absorbing nutrients, and eliminating waste, but it also houses most of our immune cells and is home to trillions of bacteria, collectively known as the microbiome. These bacteria play a crucial role in everything from mood regulation to immune defence. When the gut is healthy, it supports effective digestion, produces mood-stabilising neurotransmitters, and protects against infections.

To build a healthy gut, it's essential to eat a variety of fibre-rich foods, such as vegetables, fruits, legumes, and whole grains. Fibre acts as a prebiotic, feeding beneficial bacteria that keep the gut lining strong and support immune function. Fermented foods like yoghourt, sauerkraut, and kefir provide probiotics, which introduce beneficial bacteria to the gut, helping maintain balance and improving digestion. Reducing sugar and refined carbohydrates can also reduce inflammation and support a balanced microbiome.

## Supporting Immune Function

The immune system is constantly working to protect us from pathogens, and it relies heavily on the nutrients we consume. Building a resilient immune system requires a diet rich in vitamins, minerals, and antioxidants. Vitamin C, for example, is a powerful antioxidant found in citrus fruits, strawberries, and bell peppers that supports immune cell function. Zinc, found in nuts, seeds, and lean meats, is essential for immune cell production.

An anti-inflammatory diet, high in omega-3 fatty acids from sources like fish and flaxseed, can help reduce chronic inflammation, which is often at the root of immune dysregulation. This is why building immunity isn't just about avoiding colds and flus—it's about creating an internal environment where the body can easily ward off threats.

## Balancing Blood Sugar Levels

Stable blood sugar levels are essential for sustained energy, mental clarity, and reduced risk of chronic diseases like diabetes and heart disease. When we eat refined sugars or simple carbohydrates, blood sugar levels spike, causing a surge of insulin to manage it. Over time, frequent spikes can lead to insulin resistance, a precursor to diabetes.

Eating balanced meals with a mix of protein, fibre, and healthy fats can help stabilise blood sugar. Complex carbohydrates from whole grains, paired with proteins and fats, slow digestion and prevent rapid spikes and crashes. This balanced approach to eating keeps hunger at bay, prevents cravings, and sustains energy throughout the day.

**Fostering Mental Wellness**

Mental wellness is as much a part of health as physical wellness. Chronic stress, poor sleep, and nutrient deficiencies can contribute to mental fatigue, anxiety, and depression. Nourishing mental health starts with quality sleep, stress management techniques like meditation or exercise, and foods that support brain health. Omega-3 fatty acids, B vitamins, magnesium, and antioxidants are all key to cognitive function and emotional stability.

For example, fatty fish like salmon, nuts, and seeds are high in omega-3s, which support brain cell structure and function. Leafy greens, whole grains, and bananas are rich in B vitamins and magnesium, which play essential roles in neurotransmitter production. By incorporating foods that support the brain, we can foster mental resilience and clarity, making it easier to handle life's stresses and stay focused.

**The Path Forward**

Building health from the inside out isn't an overnight process; it's a commitment to making small, consistent changes that accumulate over time. This isn't about quick fixes or extreme diets. It's about treating food as a vital component of a broader approach to wellness—one that includes regular movement, quality sleep, and self-care practices that nurture the mind and spirit.

The LIVING GOOD DAILY COOKBOOK provides a roadmap for making this transformation achievable and enjoyable. Through recipes that focus on nutrient density, flavour, and simplicity, this book empowers you to reclaim your health one meal at a time. By shifting the focus from managing symptoms to nurturing the body with whole, nutritious foods, you're not only building resilience against disease but creating a life filled with energy, clarity, and vitality. True health care is within reach, and it starts from the inside out.

# Chapter 1: Essentials for Living Good Daily

In a world where health has become increasingly complex, it's easy to feel overwhelmed by the endless choices, conflicting advice, and quick-fix solutions surrounding us. However, true health isn't about following the latest trends or chasing temporary results—it's about creating a foundation that sustains your vitality, prevents disease, and nourishes your body for the long haul. This chapter explores the foundational principles that make up real health, including the basics of nutrition and the transformative power of whole foods and natural ingredients.

## Foundational Principles of Real Health

To achieve long-lasting health, it's essential to understand the principles that form the bedrock of well-being. These principles are not about fad diets or drastic lifestyle changes but rather about nurturing the body with a consistent and balanced approach that promotes resilience and vitality.

**Focus on Prevention, Not Reaction**

Many of us wait until we feel unwell before we consider our health, but the key to living good daily lies in a proactive approach. Rather than responding to symptoms, prevention involves maintaining a lifestyle that minimises the risk of developing chronic diseases in the first place. Prioritising whole foods, adequate hydration, physical activity, quality sleep, and stress management can help the body fend off illness and reduce the likelihood of experiencing health crises.

**Listen to Your Body**

Each person's health journey is unique, and learning to listen to your body's cues is invaluable. Your body constantly provides feedback—fatigue, headaches, digestive issues, and mood fluctuations are all signals that can indicate areas needing attention. By recognizing these signals early, you can make adjustments before minor issues become major health concerns. Building real health requires cultivating awareness and honouring your body's needs, from food and exercise to rest and relaxation.

**Create Sustainable Habits**

True health is not a quick fix; it's built on habits that can be maintained over a lifetime. Small, consistent steps are far more effective than drastic changes that are hard to maintain. Emphasising sustainability over perfection means making gradual adjustments, such as incorporating more vegetables into meals or replacing sugary drinks with water. The goal is to create a lifestyle that fits naturally into your life and provides long-term benefits without feeling restrictive.

**Prioritise Rest and Recovery**

In a fast-paced world, rest is often overlooked, yet it is one of the most crucial components of health. Quality sleep and relaxation enable the body to repair, rejuvenate, and balance hormone levels. Sleep also plays a vital role in cognitive function, memory, and mood regulation. Similarly, taking moments to unwind and practice mindfulness reduces stress, which is closely linked to numerous health conditions, including heart disease and high blood pressure.

**Embrace Whole-Person Wellness**

Wellness encompasses more than just the physical body; it includes mental, emotional, and spiritual health as well. True health is holistic, meaning it addresses the mind, body, and soul. Incorporating mental wellness practices such as mindfulness, gratitude, and self-compassion can improve emotional resilience and increase your capacity to handle stress. A strong mind-body connection is essential for lasting health and harmony in everyday life.

# Nutritional Basics for Disease Prevention

Nutrition is the cornerstone of health, and understanding its basics can empower you to make better choices for your body. Good nutrition doesn't have to be complicated; it's about providing your body with the essential nutrients it needs to function optimally and protect against illness. With a clear understanding of the basics, you can begin to harness the power of food to enhance energy, boost immunity, and prevent disease.

**Macronutrients: The Building Blocks of Health**

The body requires three primary macronutrients: carbohydrates, proteins, and fats. Each plays a unique role in maintaining health and well-being. Balancing these macronutrients can support energy levels, hormone regulation, and overall bodily functions.

Carbohydrates provide the primary fuel for the brain and muscles. Complex carbs, such as whole grains, legumes, and vegetables, release energy slowly, providing stable blood sugar levels. In contrast, refined carbs and sugars can lead to rapid spikes and crashes, contributing to inflammation and weight gain.

Proteins are essential for tissue repair, immune function, and hormone production. Choosing lean sources of protein, such as chicken, fish, legumes, and nuts, can help build and repair cells while supporting metabolic health.

Fats play a crucial role in brain health, hormone balance, and cell structure. Healthy fats, like those in olive oil, avocados, nuts, and fatty fish, are anti-inflammatory and support cardiovascular health. Avoiding trans fats and limiting saturated fats can also help reduce the risk of heart disease.

**Micronutrients: Essential Vitamins and Minerals**

Micronutrients, which include vitamins and minerals, are required in smaller amounts but are no less important for health. Deficiencies in essential nutrients can weaken the immune system, impair cognitive function, and increase the risk of chronic disease.

Vitamins such as A, C, D, and E support immune function, skin health, and energy production. B vitamins are particularly important for energy metabolism and mental clarity.

Minerals such as magnesium, calcium, iron, and zinc play roles in muscle function, bone density, and wound healing. Magnesium, for example, is essential for muscle relaxation, while calcium supports bone strength, and iron is vital for oxygen transport in the blood.

Eating a varied diet rich in colourful vegetables, fruits, whole grains, nuts, seeds, and lean proteins can help ensure you're getting a balanced range of vitamins and minerals to support your body's needs.

**Hydration: The Often-Overlooked Nutrient**

Water is perhaps the most essential yet underestimated component of a healthy diet. Proper hydration aids in digestion, circulation, temperature regulation, and detoxification. Dehydration can lead to fatigue, headaches, poor concentration, and even impair metabolism. Aim to drink water throughout the day, adjusting for factors such as physical activity, climate, and individual needs.

# The Benefits of Whole Foods and Natural Ingredients

One of the simplest and most effective ways to build health is to embrace whole foods. Whole foods undergo minimal processing, preserving their natural nutrients, fibre, and health-promoting compounds. This category includes vegetables, fruits, whole grains, nuts, seeds, legumes, and lean proteins. In contrast, processed foods often contain added sugars, unhealthy fats, artificial ingredients, and preservatives that can contribute to inflammation and disease.

**Nutrient Density Over Empty Calories**

Whole foods provide a high nutrient-to-calorie ratio, meaning they offer vitamins, minerals, and antioxidants without excessive calories. In contrast, processed foods are often calorie-dense but nutritionally poor. By choosing nutrient-dense foods, you're fueling your body with what it truly needs to function optimally, which can reduce cravings and improve energy levels.

**Dark Leafy Greens:** Rich in vitamins A, C, and K, along with fibre and folate, greens like spinach, kale, and Swiss chard promote heart health, reduce inflammation, and support brain function.

**Berries:** Loaded with antioxidants, berries like blueberries, strawberries, and raspberries protect against oxidative stress, improve skin health, and may reduce the risk of certain cancers.

**Nuts and Seeds:** Almonds, walnuts, chia seeds, and flaxseeds are packed with healthy fats, fibre, and protein, supporting heart health and providing sustained energy.

**Natural Ingredients to Reduce Inflammation**

Inflammation is the body's natural response to injury or infection, but chronic inflammation can lead to various health issues, including heart disease, arthritis, and cancer. Many whole foods contain anti-inflammatory compounds that help keep inflammation at bay.

**Turmeric:** Contains curcumin, a powerful anti-inflammatory compound known to reduce pain, improve brain health, and fight chronic inflammation.

**Ginger**: Known for its digestive and anti-inflammatory properties, ginger can relieve nausea, reduce muscle pain, and improve immune function.

**Green Tea**: High in antioxidants, green tea reduces inflammation, supports brain health, and may lower the risk of certain cancers.

**Fibre for Gut Health and Beyond**

Fibre, found abundantly in whole foods like fruits, vegetables, grains, and legumes, plays a critical role in digestive health and overall wellness. It feeds beneficial bacteria in the gut, supports healthy digestion, and helps control blood sugar levels.

**Soluble Fibre** (found in oats, apples, and beans) absorbs water and forms a gel-like substance that slows digestion, which can improve blood sugar control and lower cholesterol.

**Insoluble Fiber** (found in whole grains, nuts, and vegetables) adds bulk to stool, preventing constipation and promoting regularity.

A diet rich in fibre also supports weight management, as fibre-rich foods are filling and can reduce overall calorie intake by promoting satiety.

## Antioxidants: Protecting Cells from Damage

Oxidative stress happens when the balance between free radicals and antioxidants in the body is disrupted. Free radicals are unstable molecules that can harm cells, contributing to ageing and various diseases. Antioxidants neutralise free radicals, preventing cellular damage and reducing the risk of chronic disease.

**Vitamin C:** Found in citrus fruits, bell peppers, and broccoli, vitamin C is essential for immune health and acts as a powerful antioxidant.

**Vitamin E**: Present in nuts, seeds, and spinach, vitamin E protects cells from oxidative damage and supports skin health.

**Polyphenols:** Found in dark chocolate, green tea, and berries, polyphenols are antioxidants that protect against inflammation and improve heart health.

## Putting It All Together: Creating a Life of Health and Vitality

Building true health isn't about adhering to restrictive rules; it's about choosing foods and habits that nourish and sustain the body daily. By understanding and implementing these foundational principles, you can create a life that supports optimal health and allows you to thrive. Incorporate whole foods, pay attention to your body, stay hydrated, and prioritise rest, and you'll set a solid foundation for lifelong well-being.

# Chapter 2: Meal Planning for Lasting Health

Achieving lasting health is a journey that begins with daily choices, and meal planning is a foundational tool to help you make those choices easier. Planning meals is more than just organising food; it's a strategy for creating a balanced, nourishing lifestyle. By thoughtfully planning your meals, you can simplify healthy eating, avoid the pitfalls of convenience foods, and ensure that your body consistently receives the nutrients it needs to thrive.

## Building a Balanced Meal Plan

Creating a balanced meal plan requires an understanding of nutrition fundamentals. To fuel your body effectively, every meal should aim to include a balance of macronutrients—carbohydrates, proteins, and fats—alongside a variety of vitamins and minerals. These elements work together to support your energy levels, immune system, and overall wellness.

**Understanding Macronutrients**

Carbohydrates are the body's primary source of energy, especially for your brain and muscles. Select complex carbs such as whole grains, veggies, and legumes. These types of carbs provide fibre, which supports gut health and stabilises blood sugar.

Proteins are essential for muscle repair, immune support, and maintaining healthy hair, skin, and nails. Include a variety of protein sources, such as lean meats, poultry, fish, legumes, nuts, and seeds, to provide the essential amino acids your body needs to function well.

Fats are necessary for brain health, hormone balance, and nutrient absorption. Choose healthy fats, such as those found in olive oil, avocados, nuts, and fatty fish. These fats are anti-inflammatory and promote heart health. Try to limit your intake of unhealthy fats, like those in fried foods and heavily processed snacks.

**Including a Variety of Micronutrients**

Micronutrients like vitamins and minerals are crucial to bodily functions, from energy production to immune defence. Eating a variety of fruits and vegetables ensures that you receive a broad spectrum of these nutrients. Incorporate an array of colourful produce:

- Leafy greens like spinach and kale provide iron, calcium, and vitamin K.
- Berries are rich in antioxidants like vitamin C, which combat cellular damage.
- Cruciferous vegetables such as broccoli and cauliflower offer fibre, folate, and vitamins A, C, and E.

**Structuring Each Meal**

To sustain energy and reduce cravings, aim for a balanced combination of nutrients in each meal. Include protein for satiety, complex carbohydrates for steady energy, and healthy fats for nutrient absorption and flavor. For instance, a simple, balanced meal could look like this:

**Protein:** Grilled chicken breast or lentils.
**Carbohydrates**: Brown rice or sweet potatoes.
**Healthy fat:** Avocado slices or a handful of nuts.
**Vegetables**: A side of leafy greens or roasted carrots.

Each part of this meal contributes to satiety and long-lasting energy, creating a solid foundation for health. Structuring meals this way prevents spikes in blood sugar and minimises afternoon energy crashes.

## Tips for Preparing Real Foods with Ease

Meal planning often falters when it feels too time-consuming, but with a few practical strategies, you can prepare nutritious, whole foods without feeling overwhelmed. Here are some tips to simplify healthy cooking and meal prep:

**Batch Cooking and Freezing:** At the beginning of the week, cook large batches of staple ingredients—such as grains, proteins, and roasted vegetables. This lets you store meals or meal components in the refrigerator or freezer, making weekday meal assembly quick and easy. For example, cook a batch of brown rice, bake some chicken, or roast a sheet of vegetables to keep ready for meals over several days.

**Pre-Cut Ingredients:** Dedicate a bit of time to chopping fruits and vegetables in advance. This reduces prep time and makes it more convenient to reach for these healthy options. Diced bell peppers, onions, and carrots are great for salads, stir-fries, and scrambles. Storing prepped ingredients in airtight containers also preserves freshness.

**Utilise Time-Saving Appliances:** A slow cooker, Instant Pot, or air fryer can simplify meal preparation. These appliances require minimal hands-on time, allowing you to cook large batches of stews, grains, or roasted vegetables while you attend to other tasks. They're perfect for creating nourishing meals without the need for constant monitoring.

**Stock Essential Ingredients:** Keep a well-stocked pantry with basic items like olive oil, canned beans, whole grains, herbs, and spices. In the fridge, have versatile ingredients like eggs, leafy greens, and citrus fruits. A stocked kitchen makes it easier to prepare meals without having to run to the store.

**Embrace One-Pot and Sheet-Pan Meals:** For minimal cleanup, consider recipes that only require one pot or one pan. Meals like veggie stir-fries, grain bowls, and sheet pan dinners can be nutrient-dense while cutting down on cooking and cleanup time. Simply throw ingredients together, season, and let them cook with minimal effort.

# Creating Weekly Meal Planning Templates and Shopping Lists

With a bit of organisation, meal planning becomes second nature. A meal planning template helps you organise your thoughts and provides a simple framework to follow week after week. Use the following steps to create your own templates and shopping lists:

**Step 1: Set a Weekly Goal**

Think about the meals you want to have for the upcoming week. Plan for three main meals each day (breakfast, lunch, and dinner) and consider any snacks you may want to include. Setting a goal provides structure and helps you visualise the week ahead, ensuring a balanced variety.

**Step 2: Plan Balanced Meals**

For each day, aim to incorporate a variety of nutrients, alternating proteins, carbohydrates, and healthy fats throughout the week. For example:

**Breakfast:** Try oatmeal topped with berries and nuts, or a smoothie made with spinach, banana, and protein powder.
**Lunch:** Salad with mixed greens, chickpeas, cherry tomatoes, and a sprinkle of feta.
**Dinner:** Grilled salmon with roasted sweet potatoes and sautéed spinach.
By rotating ingredients, you introduce variety and prevent the monotony that often leads people to revert to convenience foods.

**Step 3: Make a Shopping List**

Once your weekly meal plan is set, create a shopping list. Group items into categories such as vegetables, fruits, proteins, grains, and pantry staples. This not only saves time at the store but also helps ensure you purchase everything you need for the week. When shopping, focus on whole foods rather than processed items to ensure you're fueling your body with the best ingredients.

**Step 4: Adjust Based on Your Routine**

Meal planning isn't one-size-fits-all; adapt it based on your schedule and preferences. If you know certain days are busier, choose simpler meals that require minimal prep or can be prepared in advance. This flexibility allows meal planning to fit into your lifestyle rather than feeling restrictive.

**Step 5: Maintain Consistency**

Finally, practice consistency rather than aiming for perfection. A balanced meal plan is more sustainable when it's adaptable. Life happens, and not every meal needs to be perfectly prepared. Prioritising consistency over time will yield better results and make healthy eating a natural habit.

**Putting It All Together: The Key to Lasting Health**

Meal planning is an effective tool that makes healthy eating easier, helps avoid last-minute unhealthy choices, and ensures you're nourishing your body with the nutrients it needs to thrive. By building balanced meals, preparing foods in advance, and following a structured plan, you set yourself up for lasting health.

The process may take some time to adjust to, but as you practise, it becomes second nature. The key to successful meal planning lies in understanding your body's needs, stocking your kitchen with whole, real foods, and making time for preparation. By doing so, you can confidently take control of your health, nourishing your body for the long term.

# Chapter 3: Health-Building Breakfasts

## Blueberry Chia Seed Pudding

**Ingredients:**

1 cup unsweetened almond milk

2 tbsp chia seeds

1/2 cup fresh blueberries

1/2 tsp vanilla extract

1 tsp honey or maple syrup (optional)

**Preparation:**

In a medium bowl, combine almond milk, chia seeds, vanilla extract, and honey or maple syrup (if using).

Stir thoroughly until well mixed.

Cover and refrigerate for at least 4 hours or overnight until it thickens.

Before serving, stir again and top with fresh blueberries.

**Nutritional Info (per serving):**

Calories: 150

Protein: 3g

Carbs: 15g

Fibre: 8g

Fat: 8g

# Greek Yoghourt Parfait with Mixed Berries and Nuts

**Ingredients:**

1 cup Greek yoghourt (plain, low-fat)

1/4 cup mixed berries (strawberries, blueberries, raspberries)

1 tbsp chopped almonds or walnuts

1 tsp honey (optional)

**Preparation:**

In a serving glass, get half of the Greek yoghourt layered.

Have a layer of mixed berries added over the yoghourt.

Spoon the remaining yoghourt on top.

Sprinkle chopped nuts and drizzle with honey if desired.

**Nutritional Info (per serving):**

Calories: 220

Protein: 15g

Carbs: 25g

Fibre: 4g

Fat: 7g

# Avocado Toast with Egg

**Ingredients:**

1 slice whole-grain bread

1/2 avocado, mashed

1 large egg (boiled, poached, or scrambled)

Salt and pepper, to taste

Optional: red pepper flakes or fresh herbs

**Preparation:**

Toast the whole-grain bread until golden.

Prepare the egg to your liking (boiled, poached, or scrambled).

Spread the mashed avocado on the toast.

Place the egg on top, then season with salt, pepper, and optional toppings.

**Nutritional Info (per serving):**

Calories: 250

Protein: 10g

Carbs: 18g

Fibre: 6g

Fat: 17g

# Overnight Oats with Banana and Almond Butter

**Ingredients:**

1/2 cup rolled oats

1/2 cup unsweetened almond milk

1/2 banana, sliced

1 tbsp almond butter

1 tsp chia seeds

**Preparation:**

In a jar or bowl, mix rolled oats, almond milk, and chia seeds.

Layer sliced bananas on top and drizzle almond butter over everything.

Cover and refrigerate overnight. Serve cold or warm in the morning.

**Nutritional Info (per serving):**

Calories: 300

Protein: 8g

Carbs: 40g

Fibre: 7g

Fat: 12g

# Veggie-Packed Breakfast Burrito

**Ingredients:**

1 whole-wheat tortilla

2 large eggs, whisked

1/4 cup fresh spinach, chopped

1/4 cup diced bell peppers (any colour)

2 tbsp salsa

**Preparation:**

In a pan over medium heat, scramble the eggs with spinach and diced bell peppers until cooked.

Lay the tortilla flat and spoon the egg mixture into the centre.

Add salsa on top, then wrap the tortilla like a burrito.

**Nutritional Info (per serving):**

Calories: 280

Protein: 14g

Carbs: 24g

Fibre: 5g

Fat: 14g

# Banana Spinach Smoothie

**Ingredients:**

1 ripe banana

1 cup fresh spinach

1 cup unsweetened almond milk

1 tbsp chia seeds

**Preparation:**

Place banana, spinach, almond milk, and chia seeds in a blender.

Blend until smooth and creamy.

Pour into a glass and enjoy immediately.

**Nutritional Info (per serving):**

Calories: 180

Protein: 3g

Carbs: 36g

Fibre: 7g

Fat: 4g

# Quinoa Breakfast Bowl

**Ingredients:**

1/2 cup cooked quinoa

1/4 cup mixed berries (blueberries, raspberries)

1 tbsp chopped nuts (almonds or walnuts)

1 tsp honey

**Preparation:**

In a bowl, layer cooked quinoa and mixed berries.

Sprinkle nuts on top and drizzle with honey.

Serve warm or cold.

**Nutritional Info (per serving):**

Calories: 220

Protein: 7g

Carbs: 36g

Fibre: 5g

Fat: 6g

# Sweet Potato Hash with Eggs

**Ingredients:**

1 medium sweet potato, diced

1/2 bell pepper, diced

1/4 onion, diced

2 large eggs

1 tbsp olive oil

Salt and pepper, to taste

**Preparation:**

In a skillet, have the olive oil heated over medium heat. Add sweet potato and cook until tender, about 10 minutes.

Add bell pepper and onion, cooking until soft, about 5 minutes.

Create two small wells in the mixture and crack an egg into each. Get them covered and cook until the eggs are set.

Season with salt and pepper before serving.

**Nutritional Info (per serving):**

Calories: 350

Protein: 15g

Carbs: 40g

Fibre: 7g

Fat: 14g

# Cottage Cheese with Pineapple and Flaxseed

**Ingredients:**

1 cup low-fat cottage cheese

Half cup of pineapple chunks (fresh or canned in juice)

1 tbsp ground flaxseed

**Preparation:**

In a bowl, combine cottage cheese and pineapple.

Sprinkle ground flaxseed on top.

Mix well and serve.

**Nutritional Info (per serving):**

Calories: 250

Protein: 23g

Carbs: 30g

Fibre: 3g

Fat: 5g

# Oatmeal with Almonds and Apples

**Ingredients:**

1/2 cup rolled oats

1 cup water or milk

1/2 apple, diced

1 tbsp chopped almonds

1 tsp cinnamon

1 tsp honey (optional)

**Preparation:**

In a saucepan, get either water or milk to a boil.

Add rolled oats and diced apples. Minimise the heat and simmer for about 5 minutes.

Stir in cinnamon and top with chopped almonds and honey if desired.

**Nutritional Info (per serving):**

Calories: 280

Protein: 7g

Carbs: 48g

Fibre: 7g

Fat: 8g

# Buckwheat Pancakes with Berries

**Ingredients:**

1 cup buckwheat flour

1 tbsp baking powder

1 cup almond milk

1 tbsp maple syrup

1/2 cup mixed berries

**Preparation:**

In a bowl, mix buckwheat flour and baking powder.

Add almond milk and maple syrup, stirring until smooth.

Get a skillet heated over moderate heat and pour batter to form pancakes.

Cook until bubbles form, then flip and cook until golden.

Serve topped with mixed berries.

**Nutritional Info (per serving):**

Calories: 320

Protein: 10g

Carbs: 55g

Fibre: 6g

Fat: 5g

# Savory Oatmeal with Spinach and Feta

**Ingredients:**

1/2 cup rolled oats

1 cup vegetable broth

1/2 cup fresh spinach

1/4 cup crumbled feta cheese

Salt and pepper, to taste

**Preparation:**

In a saucepan, bring vegetable broth to a boil. Add rolled oats and reduce heat, cooking until tender.

Stir in fresh spinach until wilted.

Top with crumbled feta and season with salt and pepper.

**Nutritional Info (per serving):**

Calories: 250

Protein: 11g

Carbs: 38g

Fibre: 5g

Fat: 8g

# Protein-Packed Smoothie Bowl

**Ingredients:**

1 cup spinach

1 banana

1/2 cup Greek yoghourt

1/2 cup almond milk

Toppings: sliced fruits, seeds, nuts

**Preparation:**

Blend spinach, banana, Greek yoghourt, and almond milk until smooth.

Pour into a bowl and top with sliced fruits, seeds, and nuts as desired.

**Nutritional Info (per serving):**

Calories: 300

Protein: 20g

Carbs: 40g

Fibre: 5g

Fat: 8g

# Apple Cinnamon Quinoa Bowl

**Ingredients:**

1/2 cup cooked quinoa

1/2 apple, diced

1 tsp cinnamon

1 tbsp maple syrup (optional)

1 tbsp walnuts, chopped

**Preparation:**

In a bowl, combine cooked quinoa, diced apple, and cinnamon.

Drizzle with maple syrup if desired and top with walnuts.

**Nutritional Info (per serving):**

Calories: 250

Protein: 6g

Carbs: 42g

Fibre: 6g

Fat: 10g

# Peanut Butter Banana Overnight Oats

**Ingredients:**

1/2 cup rolled oats

1 cup unsweetened almond milk

1 banana, sliced

1 tbsp peanut butter

1 tsp chia seeds

**Preparation:**

In a jar or bowl, mix rolled oats, almond milk, and chia seeds.

Layer sliced banana on top and add peanut butter.

Cover and refrigerate overnight. Serve cold.

**Nutritional Info (per serving):**

Calories: 350

Protein: 10g

Carbs: 54g

Fibre: 8g

Fat: 12g

# Chapter 4: Nourishing Lunches for Sustained Energy

## Quinoa Salad with Chickpeas and Spinach

**Ingredients:**

1 cup cooked quinoa

1 cup canned chickpeas, rinsed and drained

2 cups fresh spinach, chopped

1/2 cup cherry tomatoes, halved

1/4 cup red onion, diced

2 tbsp olive oil

1 tbsp lemon juice

Salt and pepper to taste

**Preparation:**

In a large bowl, have the cooked quinoa, chickpeas, spinach, cherry tomatoes, and red onion mixed.

In a small bowl, get the olive oil, lemon juice, salt, and pepper whisked together.

Have the dressing poured over the salad and toss to combine.

**Nutritional Info (per serving):**

Calories: 320

Protein: 12g

Carbs: 40g

Fibre: 10g

Fat: 14g

# Turkey and Avocado Wrap

**Ingredients:**

1 whole-grain wrap

4 oz turkey breast, sliced

1/2 avocado, sliced

1/2 cup lettuce

1/4 cup diced tomatoes

1 tbsp mustard

**Preparation:**

Lay the wrap flat and spread mustard over it.

Layer turkey, avocado, lettuce, and tomatoes on the wrap.

Roll tightly, slice in half, and serve.

**Nutritional Info (per serving):**

Calories: 350

Protein: 25g

Carbs: 30g

Fibre: 7g

Fat: 15g

# Mediterranean Grain Bowl

**Ingredients:**

1 cup cooked brown rice

1/2 cup cucumber, diced

1/2 cup bell pepper, diced

1/4 cup Kalamata olives, sliced

1/4 cup feta cheese, crumbled

2 tbsp olive oil

1 tbsp red wine vinegar

Salt and pepper to taste

**Preparation:**

In a bowl, combine brown rice, cucumber, bell pepper, olives, and feta cheese.

In a separate bowl, whisk together olive oil, vinegar, salt, and pepper.

Have the dressing drizzled over the bowl and toss gently to combine.

**Nutritional Info (per serving):**

Calories: 400

Protein: 12g

Carbs: 45g

Fibre: 8g

Fat: 20g

# Sweet Potato and Black Bean Tacos

**Ingredients:**

2 small sweet potatoes, peeled and diced

One cup of canned black beans, rinsed and drained

1 tsp cumin

1 tsp paprika

4 corn tortillas

1 avocado, sliced

Salsa for topping

**Preparation:**

Preheat the oven to 400°F (200°C).

Toss diced sweet potatoes with cumin and paprika, then spread on a baking sheet. Roast for about twenty-five minutes or until tender.

Warm tortillas in a skillet. Fill each with sweet potatoes, black beans, avocado, and salsa.

**Nutritional Info (per serving):**

Calories: 300

Protein: 9g

Carbs: 55g

Fibre: 15g

Fat: 10g

# Lentil Soup with Carrots and Celery

**Ingredients:**

1 cup dry lentils, rinsed

1 medium onion, chopped

2 carrots, diced

2 celery stalks, diced

4 cups vegetable broth

1 tsp thyme

Salt and pepper to taste

**Preparation:**

In a large pot, have onion, carrots, and celery sauté until softened.

Add lentils, broth, thyme, salt, and pepper. Bring to a boil.

Have the heat minimised and simmer for 30-35 minutes until lentils are tender.

**Nutritional Info (per serving):**

Calories: 230

Protein: 15g

Carbs: 40g

Fibre: 12g

Fat: 1g

# Chickpea and Avocado Salad

**Ingredients:**

1 cup canned chickpeas, rinsed and drained

1/2 avocado, diced

1/4 cup red onion, diced

1/2 cup cherry tomatoes, halved

1 tbsp lemon juice

Salt and pepper to taste

**Preparation:**

In a bowl, combine chickpeas, avocado, red onion, and cherry tomatoes. Drizzle with lemon juice, season with salt and pepper, and toss gently.

**Nutritional Info (per serving):**

Calories: 250

Protein: 10g

Carbs: 30g

Fibre: 8g

Fat: 12g

# Brown Rice Stir-Fry with Tofu

**Ingredients:**

1 cup cooked brown rice

1 cup mixed vegetables (bell pepper, broccoli, carrots)

1 cup firm tofu, cubed

2 tbsp soy sauce

1 tbsp sesame oil

1 tsp ginger, minced

**Preparation:**

Have the sesame oil heated in a pan over medium heat. Add tofu and cook until golden.

Add mixed vegetables and ginger, stir-frying for about 5 minutes.

Stir in brown rice and soy sauce, cooking until heated through.

**Nutritional Info (per serving):**

Calories: 400

Protein: 18g

Carbs: 50g

Fibre: 6g

Fat: 15g

# Egg Salad Sandwich

**Ingredients:**

4 hard-boiled eggs, chopped

2 tbsp Greek yoghourt

1 tbsp mustard

1/4 cup celery, diced

2 slices whole-grain bread

Salt and pepper to taste

**Preparation:**

In a bowl, mix chopped eggs, Greek yoghourt, mustard, celery, salt, and pepper.

Spread the egg salad on a slice of bread, top with another slice, and cut in half.

**Nutritional Info (per serving):**

Calories: 290

Protein: 20g

Carbs: 28g

Fibre: 4g

Fat: 14g

# Zucchini Noodles with Pesto and Cherry Tomatoes

**Ingredients:**

2 medium zucchinis, spiralized

1 cup cherry tomatoes, halved

1/4 cup basil pesto

1 tbsp olive oil

Salt and pepper to taste

**Preparation:**

In a skillet, have the olive oil heated over medium heat. Get the zucchini noodles added and cook for 2-3 minutes until slightly softened.

Stir in cherry tomatoes and pesto, cooking for another minute. Season with salt and pepper.

**Nutritional Info (per serving):**

Calories: 250

Protein: 4g

Carbs: 20g

Fibre: 5g

Fat: 18g

# Shrimp and Avocado Salad

**Ingredients:**

1 cup cooked shrimp

1/2 avocado, diced

1 cup mixed greens

1/4 cup red onion, thinly sliced

1 tbsp olive oil

1 tbsp lime juice

Salt and pepper to taste

**Preparation:**

In a bowl, combine shrimp, avocado, mixed greens, and red onion.

Drizzle using the olive oil and lime juice, and spice with salt and pepper.

**Nutritional Info (per serving):**

Calories: 300

Protein: 24g

Carbs: 10g

Fibre: 6g

Fat: 20g

# Roasted Vegetable and Hummus Wrap

**Ingredients:**

1 whole-grain wrap

One cup of roasted vegetables (bell peppers, zucchini, eggplant)

1/4 cup hummus

1/2 cup arugula

**Preparation:**

Spread hummus evenly over the wrap.

Layer roasted vegetables and arugula on top.

Roll tightly, slice in half, and serve.

**Nutritional Info (per serving):**

Calories: 350

Protein: 10g

Carbs: 45g

Fibre: 8g

Fat: 15g

# Tuna Salad with Beans and Corn

**Ingredients:**

1 can tuna, drained

1/2 cup canned white beans, rinsed and drained

1/2 cup corn (fresh or canned)

1/4 cup red onion, diced

2 tbsp Greek yoghourt

Salt and pepper to taste

**Preparation**:

In a bowl, combine tuna, white beans, corn, red onion, and Greek yoghourt. Spice using salt and pepper and mix well.

**Nutritional Info (per serving):**

Calories: 280

Protein: 25g

Carbs: 25g

Fibre: 6g

Fat: 8g

# Mushroom and Spinach Quinoa Bowl

**Ingredients:**

1 cup cooked quinoa

1 cup mushrooms, sliced

2 cups spinach, chopped

2 tbsp olive oil

1 garlic clove, minced

Salt and pepper to taste

**Preparation:**

In a skillet, have the olive oil heated over medium heat. Get garlic and mushrooms added, sautéing until mushrooms are browned.

Stir in spinach and cook until wilted. Mix in quinoa and season with salt and pepper.

**Nutritional Info (per serving):**

Calories: 320

Protein: 12g

Carbs: 40g

Fibre: 7g

Fat: 14g

# Baked Falafel with Tahini Sauce

**Ingredients:**

1 can chickpeas, drained and rinsed

1/4 cup onion, chopped

2 cloves garlic, minced

1 tsp cumin

1 tsp coriander

1 tbsp olive oil

1/4 cup tahini

2 tbsp lemon juice

**Preparation:**

Preheat the oven to 375°F (190°C). In a food processor, blend chickpeas, onion, garlic, cumin, coriander, and olive oil until combined. Form into small balls shapes and have them placed on a baking sheet. Bake for 25-30 minutes until golden.

In a small bowl, get the tahini, lemon juice, and water whisked together until smooth.

**Nutritional Info (per serving):**

Calories: 300

Protein: 12g

Carbs: 40g

Fibre: 10g

Fat: 12g

# Cottage Cheese Bowl with Fruits and Nuts

**Ingredients:**

1 cup cottage cheese

1/2 cup mixed berries (strawberries, blueberries, raspberries)

1 tbsp honey

2 tbsp chopped nuts (walnuts, almonds)

**Preparation:**

In a bowl, add cottage cheese and top with mixed berries, honey, and nuts.

**Nutritional Info (per serving):**

Calories: 280

Protein: 24g

Carbs: 30g

Fibre: 4g

Fat: 10g

# Chapter 5: Dinners that Heal and Restore

## Lemon Herb Grilled Chicken with Quinoa Salad

**Ingredients:**

4 chicken breasts (6 oz each)

1/4 cup olive oil

2 lemons (juiced)

2 tsp dried oregano

2 tsp garlic powder

Salt and pepper to taste

1 cup quinoa (uncooked)

2 cups water

1 cup cherry tomatoes (halved)

1 cucumber (diced)

1/4 cup parsley (chopped)

**Preparation:**

Marinate chicken in olive oil, lemon juice, oregano, garlic powder, salt, and pepper for at least 30 minutes.

Get the quinoa cooked in water according to package instructions.

Grill chicken over medium heat for 6-7 minutes per side until cooked through.

In a bowl, mix cooked quinoa, tomatoes, cucumber, and parsley. Serve with grilled chicken.

**Nutritional Info (per serving):**

Calories: 450

Protein: 37g

Carbs: 40g

Fibre: 5g

Fat: 20g

# Baked Salmon with Sweet Potato and Asparagus

**Ingredients:**

4 salmon fillets (5 oz each)

2 medium sweet potatoes (cubed)

1 lb asparagus (trimmed)

2 tbsp olive oil

2 tsp garlic powder

Salt and pepper to taste

**Preparation:**

Preheat oven to 400°F (200°C).

Toss sweet potatoes and asparagus in olive oil, garlic powder, salt, and pepper. Spread on a baking sheet.

Place salmon fillets on the sheet and season with salt and pepper. Bake for 20-25 minutes.

**Nutritional Info (per serving):**

Calories: 350

Protein: 35g

Carbs: 30g

Fibre: 8g

Fat: 15g

# Vegetable Stir-Fry with Brown Rice

**Ingredients:**

2 cups broccoli florets

1 bell pepper (sliced)

1 carrot (sliced)

1 cup snap peas

2 tbsp soy sauce (low sodium)

1 tbsp sesame oil

2 cups cooked brown rice

1/4 cup green onions (chopped)

**Preparation:**

Have the sesame oil heated in a pan over medium heat. Add vegetables and stir-fry for 5-7 minutes.

Have the soy sauce added and cook for another 2 minutes.

Serve stir-fry over brown rice and garnish using green onions.

**Nutritional Info (per serving):**

Calories: 320

Protein: 8g

Carbs: 56g

Fibre: 8g

Fat: 10g

# Quinoa-Stuffed Bell Peppers

**Ingredients:**

4 large bell peppers (any colour)

1 cup cooked quinoa

1 can black beans (rinsed and drained)

1 cup corn (canned or frozen)

1 tsp cumin

1 tsp chili powder

1 cup salsa

1/2 cup shredded cheese (optional)

**Preparation:**

Preheat oven to 375°F (190°C).

Cut the tops of the bell peppers and clear the seeds.

In a bowl, have the quinoa, black beans, corn, cumin, chili powder, and salsa mixed.

Fill peppers with the mixture, top with cheese if using, and place in a baking dish. Bake for 30 minutes.

**Nutritional Info (per serving):**

Calories: 280

Protein: 12g

Carbs: 50g

Fibre: 12g

Fat: 6g

# Lentil and Spinach Soup

**Ingredients:**

1 cup lentils (rinsed)

4 cups vegetable broth

2 cups spinach (fresh)

1 onion (chopped)

2 carrots (diced)

2 celery stalks (diced)

2 garlic cloves (minced)

1 tsp cumin

Salt and pepper to taste

**Preparation:**

In a pot, sauté onion, carrots, celery, and garlic until soft.

Add lentils, broth, cumin, salt, and pepper. Get it to a boil, then simmer for about twenty-five minutes.

Stir in spinach and cook until wilted.

**Nutritional Info (per serving):**

Calories: 220

Protein: 15g

Carbs: 36g

Fibre: 12g

Fat: 1g

# Zucchini Noodles with Tomato Basil Sauce

**Ingredients:**

4 medium zucchinis (spiralized)

2 cups cherry tomatoes (halved)

2 cloves garlic (minced)

1/4 cup fresh basil (chopped)

2 tbsp olive oil

Salt and pepper to taste

Grated Parmesan cheese (optional)

**Preparation:**

In a skillet, have the olive oil heated and sauté garlic until fragrant. Add cherry tomatoes, salt, and pepper, cooking for 5 minutes.

Stir in zucchini noodles and cook for another 3-4 minutes until tender. Add fresh basil and serve with cheese if desired.

**Nutritional Info (per serving):**

Calories: 180

Protein: 5g

Carbs: 20g

Fibre: 4g

Fat: 8g

# Chickpea Curry with Brown Rice

**Ingredients:**

1 can chickpeas (rinsed and drained)

1 can coconut milk

1 onion (chopped)

2 cloves garlic (minced)

1 tbsp curry powder

1 tsp ginger (grated)

2 cups cooked brown rice

2 cups spinach (fresh)

**Preparation:**

In a pot, get the onion and garlic sauté until soft. Add curry powder and ginger, cooking for another minute.

Stir in chickpeas and coconut milk, simmering for 15 minutes.

Add spinach until wilted. Serve over brown rice.

**Nutritional Info (per serving):**

Calories: 380

Protein: 15g

Carbs: 54g

Fibre: 10g

Fat: 14g

# Stuffed Acorn Squash

**Ingredients:**

2 acorn squashes (halved and seeds removed)

1 cup cooked quinoa

1/2 cup walnuts (chopped)

1/2 cup dried cranberries

2 tbsp maple syrup

Salt and pepper to taste

**Preparation:**

Preheat oven to 375°F (190°C).

Brush acorn squash with olive oil and sprinkle with salt and pepper. Place cut-side down on a baking sheet and bake for 30-35 minutes.

In a bowl, mix quinoa, walnuts, cranberries, and maple syrup. Have the squash turned cut-side up and fill with the mixture. Bake for another 15 minutes.

**Nutritional Info (per serving):**

Calories: 350

Protein: 10g

Carbs: 60g

Fibre: 8g

Fat: 12g

# Baked Eggplant Parmesan

**Ingredients:**

2 medium eggplants (sliced)

1 cup marinara sauce

1 cup shredded mozzarella cheese

1/2 cup grated Parmesan cheese

1/2 cup whole wheat breadcrumbs

1 tbsp Italian seasoning

Olive oil spray

**Preparation:**

Preheat oven to 375°F (190°C). Sprinkle eggplant slices with salt and let sit for 30 minutes to draw out moisture, then rinse and pat dry.

Spray a baking dish with olive oil. Layer eggplant, marinara, mozzarella, and Parmesan. Repeat layers, finishing with cheese and breadcrumbs on top.

Bake for 30-35 minutes until golden.

**Nutritional Info (per serving):**

Calories: 320

Protein: 18g

Carbs: 36g

Fibre: 10g

Fat: 12g

# Turkey and Vegetable Skillet

**Ingredients:**

1 lb ground turkey

1 zucchini (diced)

1 bell pepper (diced)

1 onion (chopped)

2 cloves garlic (minced)

1 can diced tomatoes (14 oz)

1 tsp Italian seasoning

Salt and pepper to taste

**Preparation:**

In a skillet, cook ground turkey until browned. Get the onion and garlic added, sautéing until soft.

Stir in zucchini, bell pepper, diced tomatoes, Italian seasoning, salt, and pepper. Simmer for 10-15 minutes.

**Nutritional Info (per serving):**

Calories: 350

Protein: 30g

Carbs: 20g

Fibre: 5g

Fat: 15g

# Mushroom and Spinach Risotto

**Ingredients:**

1 cup arborio rice

4 cups vegetable broth

1 cup mushrooms (sliced)

2 cups spinach (fresh)

1 onion (chopped)

2 cloves garlic (minced)

1/2 cup grated Parmesan cheese

1 tbsp olive oil

**Preparation:**

In a pot, have the olive oil heated and sauté onion and garlic until soft. Add mushrooms and cook until browned.

Stir in rice and gradually add broth, stirring constantly until absorbed.

When rice is creamy and cooked, stir in spinach and Parmesan.

**Nutritional Info (per serving):**

Calories: 420

Protein: 14g

Carbs: 65g

Fibre: 4g

Fat: 10g

# Honey-Garlic Shrimp with Broccoli

**Ingredients:**

1 lb shrimp (peeled and deveined)

2 cups broccoli florets

1/4 cup honey

3 tbsp soy sauce (low sodium)

2 cloves garlic (minced)

1 tbsp olive oil

Cooked brown rice for serving

**Preparation:**

In a bowl, mix honey, soy sauce, and garlic. Get the shrimp added and marinate for 15 minutes.

Heat olive oil in a skillet. Add broccoli and stir-fry for 3-4 minutes. Add shrimp and cook until pink, about 5 minutes.

Serve over brown rice.

**Nutritional Info (per serving):**

Calories: 350

Protein: 25g

Carbs: 40g

Fibre: 4g

Fat: 10g

# Pasta Primavera

**Ingredients:**

8 oz whole wheat pasta

1 cup cherry tomatoes (halved)

1 bell pepper (sliced)

1 zucchini (sliced)

1 carrot (sliced)

2 cloves garlic (minced)

2 tbsp olive oil

1/4 cup fresh basil (chopped)

Salt and pepper to taste

**Preparation:**

Cook pasta according to package instructions.

In a skillet, have the olive oil heated and sauté garlic and vegetables until tender.

Toss cooked pasta with vegetables, basil, salt, and pepper.

**Nutritional Info (per serving):**

Calories: 360

Protein: 12g

Carbs: 60g

Fibre: 8g

Fat: 10g

# Cauliflower Fried Rice

**Ingredients:**

1 head cauliflower (riced)

2 eggs (beaten)

1 cup mixed vegetables (carrots, peas, corn)

2 green onions (chopped)

2 tbsp soy sauce (low sodium)

1 tbsp sesame oil

Salt and pepper to taste

**Preparation:**

In a pan, heat sesame oil and scramble the eggs. Remove and set aside.

Sauté mixed vegetables in the same pan until tender.

Add riced cauliflower, soy sauce, and cooked eggs, stir-frying for 5-7 minutes.

**Nutritional Info (per serving):**

Calories: 220

Protein: 10g

Carbs: 18g

Fibre: 5g

Fat: 12g

# Balsamic Glazed Brussels Sprouts and Carrots

**Ingredients:**

2 cups Brussels sprouts (halved)

2 cups carrots (sliced)

1/4 cup balsamic vinegar

2 tbsp olive oil

Salt and pepper to taste

**Preparation:**

Preheat oven to 400°F (200°C). Toss Brussels sprouts and carrots with olive oil, balsamic vinegar, salt, and pepper.

Get them spread on a baking sheet and roast for 20-25 minutes until tender.

**Nutritional Info (per serving):**

Calories: 180

Protein: 4g

Carbs: 30g

Fibre: 10g

Fat: 8g

# Chapter 6: Desserts and Snacks for Real Health

## Chia Seed Pudding

**Ingredients:**

1/2 cup chia seeds

2 cups almond milk (unsweetened)

2 tbsp maple syrup

1 tsp vanilla extract

Fresh berries for topping

**Preparation:**

In a bowl, get the chia seeds, almond milk, maple syrup, and vanilla extract whisked together.

Refrigerate for either about four hours or overnight until it thickens.

Serve with fresh berries on top.

**Nutritional Info (per serving):**

Calories: 210

Protein: 5g

Carbs: 25g

Fibre: 10g

Fat: 10g

# Avocado Chocolate Mousse

**Ingredients:**

2 ripe avocados

1/2 cup cocoa powder

1/2 cup maple syrup

1/4 cup almond milk

1 tsp vanilla extract

**Preparation:**

In a blender, have all the ingredients combined and blend until smooth.

Chill in the refrigerator for about thirty minutes, then serve.

**Nutritional Info (per serving):**

Calories: 180

Protein: 3g

Carbs: 23g

Fibre: 8g

Fat: 9g

# Oatmeal Energy Bites

**Ingredients:**

1 cup rolled oats

1/2 cup almond butter

1/4 cup honey

1/4 cup chocolate chips

1/4 cup flaxseed meal

**Preparation:**

In a bowl, have all the ingredients mixed until combined.

Roll into small balls and refrigerate for about thirty minutes.

**Nutritional Info (per serving, 2 bites):**

Calories: 220

Protein: 6g

Carbs: 30g

Fibre: 5g

Fat: 10g

# Banana Ice Cream

**Ingredients:**

2 ripe bananas, sliced and frozen

1 tbsp peanut butter (optional)

1/2 tsp vanilla extract

**Preparation:**

In a food processor, have the frozen bananas blended until smooth and creamy.

Add peanut butter and vanilla extract, blending until combined. Serve immediately.

**Nutritional Info (per serving):**

Calories: 105

Protein: 1g

Carbs: 27g

Fibre: 3g

Fat: 0g (add 3g for peanut butter)

# Almond Flour Chocolate Chip Cookies

**Ingredients:**

2 cups almond flour

1/2 tsp baking soda

1/4 cup coconut oil (melted)

1/4 cup maple syrup

1/2 cup dark chocolate chips

**Preparation:**

Preheat oven to 350°F (175°C).

In a bowl, mix almond flour and baking soda. In another bowl, get the melted coconut oil and maple syrup combined.

Mix the wet and dry ingredients, then fold in chocolate chips.

Scoop onto a baking sheet and bake for about twelve minutes.

**Nutritional Info (per cookie, makes 12):**

Calories: 140

Protein: 3g

Carbs: 10g

Fibre: 2g

Fat: 10g

# Greek Yoghourt Parfait

**Ingredients:**

1 cup Greek yoghourt (plain, unsweetened)

1/2 cup granola (low sugar)

1/2 cup mixed berries (blueberries, strawberries)

**Preparation:**

In a glass, get the Greek yogurt, granola, and berries layered.

Repeat the layers until ingredients are used up. Serve immediately.

**Nutritional Info (per serving):**

Calories: 300

Protein: 20g

Carbs: 40g

Fibre: 5g

Fat: 5g

# Coconut Macaroons

**Ingredients:**

3 cups shredded coconut (unsweetened)

1/2 cup almond flour

1/3 cup honey

2 egg whites

1 tsp vanilla extract

**Preparation:**

Preheat oven to 325°F (160°C).

In a bowl, get all the ingredients combined until mixed well.

Form small mounds and place on a baking sheet. Bake for 15-20 minutes until golden.

**Nutritional Info (per macaroon, makes 12):**

Calories: 130

Protein: 2g

Carbs: 10g

Fibre: 2g

Fat: 9g

# Sweet Potato Brownies

**Ingredients:**

1 cup mashed sweet potatoes (cooked)

1/2 cup almond flour

1/4 cup cocoa powder

1/4 cup maple syrup

1/4 cup dark chocolate chips

1 tsp vanilla extract

**Preparation:**

Preheat oven to 350°F (175°C).

In a bowl, get all the ingredients mixed until combined.

Pour into a greased baking dish and bake for 25-30 minutes.

**Nutritional Info (per brownie, makes 12):**

Calories: 140

Protein: 3g

Carbs: 23g

Fibre: 3g

Fat: 5g

# Berry Coconut Popsicles

**Ingredients:**

2 cups mixed berries (fresh or frozen)

1 cup coconut milk (full-fat)

2 tbsp honey (optional)

**Preparation:**

Blend all ingredients until smooth.

Get it poured into popsicle moulds and freeze for at least 4 hours.

**Nutritional Info (per popsicle, makes 6):**

Calories: 60

Protein: 1g

Carbs: 15g

Fibre: 3g

Fat: 2g

# Dark Chocolate Dipped Fruit

**Ingredients:**

One cup of strawberries (or any fruit of choice)

1 cup dark chocolate chips

1 tbsp coconut oil

**Preparation:**

Get the dark chocolate and coconut oil melted together in a microwave or double boiler.

Dip fruit into melted chocolate and place on parchment paper. Refrigerate until set.

**Nutritional Info (per serving, 2 strawberries):**

Calories: 150

Protein: 1g

Carbs: 20g

Fibre: 3g

Fat: 7g

# Pumpkin Spice Energy Bites

**Ingredients:**

1 cup rolled oats

1/2 cup pumpkin puree

1/4 cup honey

1/4 cup almond butter

1 tsp pumpkin spice

**Preparation:**

In a bowl, get all the ingredients until well combined.

Roll into small balls and have them refrigerated for 30 minutes.

**Nutritional Info (per serving, 2 bites):**

Calories: 180

Protein: 5g

Carbs: 28g

Fibre: 4g

Fat: 6g

# Lemon Almond Energy Balls

**Ingredients:**

1 cup almonds (raw)

1 cup pitted dates

Zest of 1 lemon

2 tbsp lemon juice

1/4 tsp salt

**Preparation:**

In a food processor, blend all ingredients until finely chopped and sticky.

Roll into small balls and have them refrigerated for 30 minutes.

**Nutritional Info (per serving, 2 balls):**

Calories: 200

Protein: 5g

Carbs: 28g

Fibre: 4g

Fat: 9g

# Apple Nachos

**Ingredients:**

2 medium apples (sliced)

2 tbsp almond butter

2 tbsp granola

1 tbsp dark chocolate chips

**Preparation:**

Arrange apple slices on a plate.

Drizzle almond butter on top, then sprinkle granola and chocolate chips.

**Nutritional Info (per serving):**

Calories: 250

Protein: 4g

Carbs: 35g

Fibre: 6g

Fat: 12g

# Nut Butter Banana Bites

**Ingredients:**

2 bananas (sliced)

1/4 cup almond butter

1/4 cup shredded coconut (unsweetened)

**Preparation:**

Spread almond butter on each banana slice.

Sprinkle shredded coconut on top. Serve immediately.

**Nutritional Info (per serving, 2 bites):**

Calories: 200

Protein: 4g

Carbs: 30g

Fibre: 4g

Fat: 8g

# Homemade Granola Bars

**Ingredients:**

2 cups rolled oats

1/2 cup almond butter

1/4 cup honey

1/4 cup mixed nuts (chopped)

1/4 cup dried fruit (raisins, cranberries)

**Preparation:**

Preheat oven to 350°F (175°C) and line a baking dish with parchment paper.

Get all ingredients mixed in a bowl until thoroughly combined.

Press mixture into the baking dish and bake for 15-20 minutes.

Allow to cool before cutting into bars.

**Nutritional Info (per bar, makes 10):**

Calories: 180

Protein: 5g

Carbs: 24g

Fibre: 3g

Fat: 8g

# Chapter 7: Supercharged Smoothies and Juices

## Green Power Smoothie

**Ingredients:**

1 cup spinach

1 banana

1/2 cup pineapple chunks (fresh or frozen)

1/2 cup almond milk (unsweetened)

1 tablespoon chia seeds

**Preparation:**

Place all ingredients in a blender.

Blend on high until smooth. If it's too thick, get a little more almond milk added.

**Nutritional Info (per serving):**

Calories: 210

Protein: 4g

Carbs: 37g

Fibre: 7g

Fat: 6g

# Berry Blast Smoothie

**Ingredients:**

1 cup mixed berries (strawberries, blueberries, raspberries)

1/2 cup Greek yoghourt (plain, unsweetened)

1 tablespoon honey

1 cup almond milk

**Preparation:**

Combine all ingredients in a blender.

Blend until smooth and creamy.

**Nutritional Info (per serving):**

Calories: 220

Protein: 10g

Carbs: 34g

Fibre: 5g

Fat: 5g

# Tropical Mango Smoothie

**Ingredients:**

1 cup mango chunks (fresh or frozen)

1 banana

1 cup coconut water

1 tablespoon flaxseed meal

**Preparation:**

Add all ingredients to a blender.

Blend until smooth and enjoy!

**Nutritional Info (per serving):**

Calories: 190

Protein: 2g

Carbs: 46g

Fibre: 5g

Fat: 1g

# Chocolate Peanut Butter Smoothie

**Ingredients:**

1 banana

1 tablespoon cocoa powder

2 tablespoons peanut butter

1 cup almond milk

1 tablespoon honey (optional)

**Preparation:**

In a blender, combine all ingredients.

Blend until smooth and creamy.

**Nutritional Info (per serving):**

Calories: 320

Protein: 8g

Carbs: 30g

Fibre: 4g

Fat: 18g

# Avocado Spinach Smoothie

**Ingredients:**

1/2 avocado

1 cup spinach

1 banana

1 cup almond milk

1 tablespoon lime juice

**Preparation:**

Combine all ingredients in a blender.

Blend until smooth and creamy.

**Nutritional Info (per serving):**

Calories: 230

Protein: 4g

Carbs: 28g

Fibre: 10g

Fat: 12g

# Cucumber Mint Juice

**Ingredients:**

1 large cucumber, peeled and chopped

1/2 cup fresh mint leaves

1 tablespoon lime juice

1-2 teaspoons honey (optional)

1 cup water

**Preparation:**

Blend all ingredients until smooth.

Strain through a fine mesh sieve or cheesecloth to remove pulp if desired.

**Nutritional Info (per serving):**

Calories: 40

Protein: 1g

Carbs: 10g

Fibre: 1g

Fat: 0g

# Beetroot Berry Smoothie

**Ingredients:**

1 small cooked beetroot

1/2 cup mixed berries

1/2 banana

1 cup almond milk

1 tablespoon chia seeds

**Preparation:**

Place all ingredients in a blender.

Blend until smooth and creamy.

**Nutritional Info (per serving):**

Calories: 200

Protein: 4g

Carbs: 40g

Fibre: 8g

Fat: 6g

# Pineapple Green Juice

**Ingredients:**

1 cup fresh pineapple chunks

2 cups kale or spinach

1 cucumber

1/2 lemon (juiced)

1 cup water

**Preparation:**

Blend all ingredients until smooth.

Strain if desired, or enjoy as a pulp-rich juice.

**Nutritional Info (per serving):**

Calories: 80

Protein: 2g

Carbs: 20g

Fibre: 2g

Fat: 0g

# Coconut Banana Smoothie

**Ingredients:**

1 banana

1 cup coconut milk (unsweetened)

1 tablespoon shredded coconut (unsweetened)

1 tablespoon honey (optional)

**Preparation:**

In a blender, combine all ingredients.

Blend until smooth and creamy.

**Nutritional Info (per serving):**

Calories: 210

Protein: 2g

Carbs: 30g

Fibre: 3g

Fat: 9g

# Carrot Ginger Juice

**Ingredients:**

3 medium carrots, peeled and chopped

1-inch piece of fresh ginger

1 apple, cored and chopped

1 cup water

**Preparation:**

Blend all ingredients until smooth.

Strain if desired, or enjoy as a pulp-rich juice.

**Nutritional Info (per serving):**

Calories: 90

Protein: 1g

Carbs: 22g

Fibre: 2g

Fat: 0g

# Orange Turmeric Smoothie

**Ingredients:**

2 oranges, peeled and segmented

1/2 banana

1 teaspoon fresh turmeric (or 1/4 teaspoon powdered)

1 cup almond milk

1 tablespoon honey (optional)

**Preparation:**

Combine all ingredients in a blender.

Blend until smooth and enjoy!

**Nutritional Info (per serving):**

Calories: 180

Protein: 2g

Carbs: 45g

Fibre: 4g

Fat: 2g

# Apple Cinnamon Smoothie

**Ingredients:**

1 apple, cored and chopped

1 banana

1/2 teaspoon ground cinnamon

1 cup almond milk

1 tablespoon almond butter

**Preparation:**

In a blender, combine all ingredients.

Blend until smooth and creamy.

**Nutritional Info (per serving):**

Calories: 250

Protein: 6g

Carbs: 38g

Fibre: 6g

Fat: 9g

# Spinach Avocado Smoothie

**Ingredients:**

1 cup spinach

1/2 avocado

1 banana

1 cup coconut water

1 tablespoon lime juice

**Preparation:**

Combine all ingredients in a blender.

Blend until smooth and creamy.

**Nutritional Info (per serving):**

Calories: 260

Protein: 4g

Carbs: 30g

Fibre: 10g

Fat: 15g

# Strawberry Basil Juice

**Ingredients:**

1 cup strawberries (fresh or frozen)

1/2 cup basil leaves

1 tablespoon lemon juice

1 cup water

**Preparation:**

Blend all ingredients until smooth.

Strain if desired, or enjoy as a pulp-rich juice.

**Nutritional Info (per serving):**

Calories: 60

Protein: 1g

Carbs: 15g

Fibre: 2g

Fat: 0g

# Peach Green Smoothie

**Ingredients:**

1 ripe peach (pitted and chopped)

1 cup spinach

1/2 cup Greek yoghourt (plain, unsweetened)

1 cup almond milk

1 tablespoon flaxseed meal

**Preparation:**

Place all ingredients in a blender.

Blend until smooth and creamy.

**Nutritional Info (per serving):**

Calories: 210

Protein: 8g

Carbs: 30g

Fibre: 6g

Fat: 6g

# Chapter 8: 30-Day Meal Plan (Bonus 1)

## Day 1 to 7

**Day 1**

Breakfast: Blueberry Chia Seed Pudding

Lunch: Quinoa Salad with Black Beans and Avocado

Dinner: Grilled Lemon Herb Chicken with Steamed Broccoli

Snack: Dark Chocolate Avocado Mousse

**Day 2**

Breakfast: Spinach and Feta Omelette

Lunch: Lentil Soup with Carrots and Celery

Dinner: Baked Salmon with Asparagus

Snack: Almond Butter and Banana on Rice Cakes

**Day 3**

Breakfast: Oatmeal with Fresh Berries and Nuts

Lunch: Mediterranean Chickpea Salad

Dinner: Stir-Fried Tofu with Vegetables

Snack: Hummus with Carrot Sticks

**Day 4**

Breakfast: Banana Pancakes with Maple Syrup

Lunch: Turkey and Avocado Wrap

Dinner: Stuffed Bell Peppers with Quinoa and Black Beans

Snack: Greek Yoghourt with Honey and Walnuts

**Day 5**

Breakfast: Green Smoothie with Spinach and Banana

Lunch: Vegetable Stir-Fry with Brown Rice

Dinner: Lemon Garlic Shrimp with Zucchini Noodles

Snack: Apple Slices with Peanut Butter

**Day 6**

Breakfast: Overnight Oats with Chia Seeds and Almond Milk

Lunch: Spinach Salad with Grilled Chicken

Dinner: Beef and Broccoli Stir-Fry

Snack: Energy Bites with Dates and Nuts

**Day 7**

Breakfast: Smoothie Bowl with Mixed Berries and Granola

Lunch: Caprese Salad with Fresh Basil

Dinner: Baked Cod with a Tomato Basil Sauce

Snack: Trail Mix with Nuts and Dried Fruits

# Day 8 to 14

**Day 8**

Breakfast: Avocado Toast with Poached Egg

Lunch: Roasted Vegetable Quinoa Bowl

Dinner: Chicken Fajitas with Bell Peppers

Snack: Coconut Macaroons

**Day 9**

Breakfast: Apple Cinnamon Oatmeal

Lunch: Asian Chicken Salad with Sesame Dressing

Dinner: Spaghetti Squash with Marinara Sauce

Snack: Dark Chocolate-Covered Almonds

**Day 10**

Breakfast: Smoothie with Kale, Pineapple, and Ginger

Lunch: Tomato Basil Soup with Whole Grain Bread

Dinner: Grilled Pork Chops with Sweet Potato Mash

Snack: Yogurt Parfait with Berries and Granola

**Day 11**

Breakfast: Scrambled Eggs with Tomatoes and Spinach

Lunch: Quinoa and Roasted Beet Salad

Dinner: Moroccan Chickpea Stew

Snack: Sliced Cucumbers with Tzatziki Sauce

**Day 12**

Breakfast: Mixed Berry Smoothie

Lunch: Chicken Caesar Salad with Whole Wheat Croutons

Dinner: Stuffed Zucchini Boats

Snack: Homemade Fruit Leather

**Day 13**

Breakfast: Nut Butter Smoothie with Bananas

Lunch: Roasted Cauliflower and Chickpea Bowl

Dinner: Grilled Lemon Rosemary Chicken

Snack: Fresh Fruit Salad

**Day 14**

Breakfast: Quinoa Breakfast Bowl with Almonds and Berries

Lunch: Taco Salad with Ground Turkey

Dinner: Pan-Seared Tilapia with Green Beans

Snack: Rice Cakes with Cream Cheese and Chives

# Day 15 to 21

**Day 15**

Breakfast: Raspberry Chia Pudding

Lunch: Mediterranean Couscous Salad

Dinner: Vegetable Curry with Brown Rice

Snack: Baked Sweet Potato Chips

**Day 16**

Breakfast: Smoothie with Spinach, Mango, and Coconut Milk

Lunch: Buffalo Chicken Wrap with Lettuce

Dinner: Beef Tacos with Fresh Salsa

Snack: Roasted Chickpeas

**Day 17**

Breakfast: Oatmeal with Peanut Butter and Banana

Lunch: Caprese Quinoa Bowl

Dinner: Lemon Herb Grilled Chicken Thighs

Snack: Dark Chocolate Energy Balls

**Day 18**

Breakfast: Protein Pancakes with Maple Syrup

Lunch: Black Bean Soup with Avocado

Dinner: Salmon Cakes with Mixed Greens

Snack: Celery Sticks with Almond Butter

**Day 19**

Breakfast: Tropical Smoothie Bowl

Lunch: Greek Salad with Feta and Olives

Dinner: Stuffed Acorn Squash with Quinoa

Snack: Dried Apricots and Walnuts

**Day 20**

Breakfast: Egg and Veggie Breakfast Muffins

Lunch: Chicken and Broccoli Stir-Fry

Dinner: Shrimp Tacos with Cabbage Slaw

Snack: Sliced Apples with Cheddar Cheese

**Day 21**

Breakfast: Green Protein Smoothie

Lunch: Sweet Potato and Black Bean Salad

Dinner: Grilled Steak with Roasted Vegetables

Snack: Chia Seed Pudding

# Day 22 to 30

**Day 22**

Breakfast: Peanut Butter Banana Overnight Oats

Lunch: Quinoa Salad with Grapes and Walnuts

Dinner: Zucchini Noodles with Pesto

Snack: Almond Joy Energy Bites

**Day 23**

Breakfast: Yogurt with Granola and Fresh Fruit

Lunch: Tuna Salad with Chickpeas

Dinner: Stuffed Bell Peppers with Ground Turkey

Snack: Guacamole with Tortilla Chips

**Day 24**

Breakfast: Coconut Mango Smoothie

Lunch: Falafel Wrap with Tahini Sauce

Dinner: Baked Chicken Thighs with Sweet Potatoes

Snack: Fruit and Nut Mix

**Day 25**

Breakfast: Overnight Oats with Almond Milk and Chia

Lunch: Spinach and Feta Stuffed Chicken Breast

Dinner: Thai Red Curry with Tofu

Snack: Banana Oatmeal Cookies

**Day 26**

Breakfast: Berry Almond Smoothie

Lunch: Mixed Green Salad with Grilled Salmon

Dinner: Veggie Stir-Fry with Cashew Sauce

Snack: Chocolate-Dipped Strawberries

**Day 27**

Breakfast: Pumpkin Spice Overnight Oats

Lunch: Lentil and Spinach Salad

Dinner: Grilled Mahi Mahi with Quinoa

Snack: Spiced Nuts

**Day 28**

Breakfast: Chocolate Banana Smoothie

Lunch: Caesar Salad with Shrimp

Dinner: Chicken and Vegetable Skewers

Snack: Fruit Smoothie

**Day 29**

Breakfast: Green Smoothie with Spinach and Pear

Lunch: Roasted Beet and Goat Cheese Salad

Dinner: Pork Tenderloin with Roasted Carrots

Snack: Greek Yoghourt with Honey

**Day 30**

Breakfast: Chia Seed Pudding with Mixed Berries

Lunch: Quinoa Tabbouleh with Grilled Chicken

Dinner: Baked Eggplant Parmesan

Snack: Rice Cakes with Almond Butter

# Conclusion: Living Good Daily Beyond the Kitchen

As we conclude our exploration of a lifestyle centred on health and nourishment, it becomes clear that the journey toward optimal wellness extends far beyond the recipes crafted in the kitchen. The principles discussed throughout this book lay a solid foundation for a holistic approach to living good daily. This conclusion will delve into the essential aspects of sustaining healthy habits, understanding the mind-body connection, and providing encouragement for your health-building journey.

## Healthy Habits for a Lifetime

Adopting a healthy lifestyle is not just a fleeting trend; it is a commitment to oneself that promises lifelong benefits. Developing healthy habits can significantly improve physical health, mental well-being, and overall quality of life. Start with small, manageable changes that can easily be integrated into daily routines. This could mean choosing whole foods over processed options, incorporating more fruits and vegetables into your meals, or making a conscious effort to stay hydrated throughout the day.

Furthermore, establishing a consistent physical activity regimen is crucial. Aim for at least 150 minutes of moderate aerobic exercise weekly, combined with strength training exercises at least two days a week. Whether it's brisk walking, cycling, yoga, or dance, find activities that you enjoy, as this will make it easier to stay committed. Keep in mind, the aim is progress, not perfection. Celebrate your small victories and understand that every step you take towards a healthier lifestyle counts.

Another key component of healthy habits is mindfulness and self-care. Prioritise getting enough sleep, as it is essential for recovery and mental clarity. Create a calming nighttime routine that prepares your body and mind for rest. Engaging in mindfulness practices, such as meditation or deep breathing exercises, can also enhance mental well-being and reduce stress. By cultivating these healthy habits, you not only support your physical health but also nurture your emotional and mental states.

# The Mind-Body Connection in Health

The mind-body connection is a powerful aspect of overall health that often gets overlooked. Our thoughts, feelings, and beliefs significantly impact our physical well-being. Negative emotions and chronic stress can lead to inflammation, weakened immune function, and various chronic diseases. Conversely, positive thoughts and emotional resilience can bolster health and enhance recovery from illness.

Practising mindfulness and self-awareness can strengthen this connection. Mindfulness encourages individuals to live in the moment, acknowledging thoughts and feelings without judgement. This practice can reduce stress and anxiety, leading to better health outcomes. Incorporating activities that promote mental health, such as journaling, yoga, or engaging in creative hobbies, can further enhance this connection.

Additionally, the value of social connections is immeasurable. Surrounding yourself with supportive friends and family can foster a sense of belonging and purpose, significantly impacting mental health. Seek to cultivate meaningful relationships and engage in community activities. These connections provide emotional support, which is vital for maintaining motivation and commitment to a healthy lifestyle.

# Encouragement for the Health-Building Journey

Embarking on a health-building journey is a deeply personal experience, and it's important to remember that it's not a linear path. You may encounter obstacles along the way, and there may be times when progress feels slow. During these moments, it's crucial to remain patient and kind to yourself. Every effort counts, and every healthy choice is a step toward a better you.

Remember that your health journey is unique. Compare your progress to your own past experiences rather than to others. Set realistic goals that resonate with your personal values and desires. Whether it's reducing stress, increasing energy levels, or improving your overall health, keep these goals at the forefront of your journey.

Celebrate milestones, no matter how small. Reward yourself for sticking to your meal plans, completing a challenging workout, or simply choosing to prioritise self-care. These celebrations act as encouragement to continue progressing.

In conclusion, living good daily is a holistic approach that encompasses much more than diet alone. It involves cultivating healthy habits, recognizing the profound connection between mind and body, and fostering resilience and encouragement throughout your journey. As you take the lessons learned from this book into your daily life, remember that every step you take towards health is a step towards a vibrant, fulfilling life. Embrace the journey and know that a healthier, happier you is not just a destination but a way of living.

# 4 BOOKS BONUS GIFTS

Please scan each QR code one by one, and you'll be directed to a website where you can claim your free books. Whenever you're prompted to enter a price, simply input "$0," as these books are completely free for you.

## BONUS 2
### 50 JUICES

## BONUS 3
### 50 SMOOTHIES

## BONUS 4
### 50 SNACKS

## BONUS 5
### 50 DESSERTS

Made in the USA
Monee, IL
06 December 2024